HOMEMADE MEDICAL FACE MASKS

The definitive guide to Make at Home 5 Different Types of Face Masks Easy explanation, Step by step with illustration.

Gabriel Reed

assurance. The trademarks that are used are without any consent, and the publication of the trademark is without permission or backing by the trademark owner. All trademarks and brands within this book are for clarifying purposes only and are the owned by the owners themselves, not affiliated with this document.

Disclaimer

Please note the information contained within this document is for education and entertainment purpose only. All effort has been executed to present accurate, up to date, reliable, complete information. No warranties of any kind are declared or implied. Readers acknowledge that the author is not engaged in the rendering of legal, financial, medical or professional advice. The content within this book has been derived from various sources. Please consult a licensed professional before attempting any techniques outlined in this book.

Table of Contents

3

How to create an effective homemade mask   **32**

INTRODUCTION

I n recent years Humanity is experiencing a real environmental crisis, the entire planet is facing a problem of enormous dimensions with devastating effects on the lives of all human beings, namely the pollution of natural resources.

This phenomenon is very often underestimated by the majority of the population who does not realize the gravity of the problem and the countless and inevitable consequences triggered by the destruction of the earth's environment. Air pollution damages the environment and human health, moreover it can cause various lung diseases and respiratory problems. A significant part of the world's population lives in areas, particularly in cities, where air quality standards are exceeded: pollution by ozone, nitrogen dioxide and particulate matters pose serious health risks. As if that wasn't enough, one of the triggers of infectious diseases can always be traced back to a critical condition of the balance between man and nature.

Some examples are relatively recent, such as bovine spongiform encephalopathy (Bovine spongiform encephalopathy (BSE) in 2000, SARS in 2002 and the avian influenza epidemic in 2003.

In January 2020, a new contagious and potentially fatal coronavirus was declared in China.

Only one month later, the epidemic has already taken on exceptional proportions. The first one thousand deaths are counted and the contagion has spread to more than fifty countries outside China. These are just initial data on this pandemic that is affecting the whole world. Unfortunately, it is virtually impossible to ignore air pollution, just as it is very difficult to contain the spread of infectious diseases and their effects, but we can save ourselves by using preventive measures such as the face mask.

A face mask doesn't only protect against air pollution and respiratory diseases but also helps to protect us from the many pathogens around us. Most diseases are transmitted from person to person through coughing and sneezing droplets, and sometimes through the steam coming out from our mouths when we speak. These tiny droplets have pathogens that remain in the air for quite a long time. A face mask prevents these droplets from remaining in the air if one person coughs or sneezes and protects others who might otherwise become infected. Using a face mask will protect us from microorganisms that can cause a variety of respiratory diseases, from a simple flu to more complex and often fatal diseases.

In addition, as the level of toxic gases increases in the environment due to human activities, a face mask will protect us and save us from chronic diseases such as asthma or bronchitis.

If we wear a protective measure such as a face mask, we will be safe somehow. Facial masks are also useful for workers working in mines, firefighters and all those people who are often forced to work in hazardous environmental conditions. In our daily life, a face mask is always useful because it protects us from most airborne diseases. It is true that face masks are on the market but learning how to make your own face mask at home will help you in emergency situations like the one we are experiencing now. Coronavirus has triggered fears of contagion and you don't stop running to buy one.

Being able to make a face mask can save you time and money, and you can also create masks for your family and friends. You can customize them in terms of beauty but above all in terms of safety according to the use you will have to make them. Face masks are recommended by the World Health Organization, CDC as protective gears. However, there may be situations where facial masks may be constantly sold out in pharmacies, markets, or the price may be high due to black marketing.

Therefore, it is useful to be able to make our Facial Mask yourself at home and use this ability in case of emergency. In this article, we will learn how to make different varieties of facial masks at home using the items already present in our home. We will also find out when it is useful to wear a facial mask, the correct ways to wear it and remove it after use. We will know the effectiveness of homemade face masks.

1

HOWEMADE MEDICAL FACE MASKS

In many workplaces, personnel find themselves operating in the presence of aerosols and fine dust. The latters are usually referred to as PMx, where x indicates the particle size expressed in μm.

When we talk about aerosols and particulate matter we are referring to systems which, regardless of their chemical composition, have very variable dimensions. If they are between 2 nm and 2 μm we are dealing with colloidal systems that remain dispersed in the air due to their size. Thanks to them, in fact, the force of gravity is not able to prevail over dispersive forces such as, for example, repulsion between electric charges or interactions with air molecules.

As a consequence, these particles remain dispersed in the air until factors, that allow the force of gravity to predominate and permit their deposition on the ground, intervene. To give you an idea of what the numbers written above mean, keep in mind that nm (read nanometer) corresponds to one billionth of a meter, while µm (read micrometer) corresponds to one millionth of a meter. Considering that the length of a chemical bond, such as the C-H bond, is about 0.1 nm, the result is that 2 nm is a dimension that corresponds to about 20 times the carbon-hydrogen distance, while 2 µm corresponds to about 20000 times the same distance. That still doesn't tell you anything, does it? In fact, if you haven't studied chemistry, you can not realize how small a chemical bond is.

Then let's look at the picture in Figure 1.

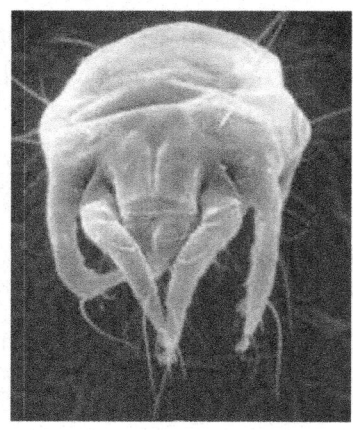

Figure 1

It is a dust mite whose size is about 0.5 mm, which is about 250 times larger than 2 μm and represents the upper limit of the size range into which the colloidal particles fall. The photo in Figure 1 was obtained under an electron microscope.

In other words, dust mites are not visible to the naked eye. You can now easily imagine that colloidal particles are not visible to the naked eye either. You could say to me, "What are you saying? That's not true. I can see the smog particles." (these in the common imagination are understood as fine dust).

I am sorry to inform you that the particles that you see with the naked eye are much larger than those in the range 2 nm-2 μm (let's say at least more than 1000 times larger), while the particles whose size falls in the above range cannot be seen except by electron microscopy. When the particles are so small, the only visible effect is the one that goes under the name "Tyndall effect".

In practice, the light that "meets" the colloidal particles is dispersed in all directions (Figure 2) with the consequence that a solution appears opaque or the air appears "nebulous".

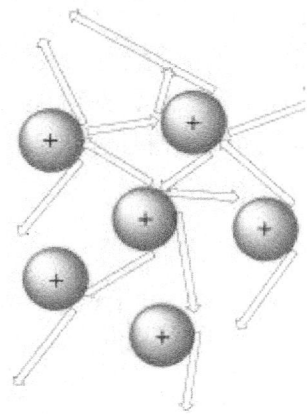

Figure 2

BUT WHAT DOES THAT HAVE TO DO WITH FILTER MASKS?

As I said, in many workplaces, staff come into contact with particulate matter. These are very dangerous for us since they can trigger many pathologies, first of all respiratory ones. Employers are therefore obliged to provide their employees with personal protective equipment, including masks. These are able to filter the fine dust in the air and prevent it from being inhaled.

There are different types of filter masks that are indicated by their initials:

TYPE FFP1/P1

Protection from non-toxic and non-fibrogenic dust

Inhalation does not cause the development of diseases; however, it can irritate the respiratory tract and represent odor pollution.

The total loss may be a maximum of 25%.

The occupational exposure limit value may be exceeded by a maximum of 4 times.

Respiratory masks of protection class FFP1 are suitable for working environments where toxic or fibrogenic dusts and aerosols are not expected. They filter at least 80% of the particles in the air up to a size of 0.6 µm and can be used when the occupational exposure limit value is not exceeded by more than 4 times. In the construction or food industry, respiratory masks of class FFP1 are almost always sufficient.

TYPE FFP2/P2/N95

Protection from dust, smoke and aerosol solids and liquids harmful to health

The particles may be fibrogenic, i.e. in the short term they cause irritation of the respiratory tract and in the long term they lead to a reduction in the elasticity of lung tissue

The total loss may be a maximum of 11%.

The occupational exposure limit value may be exceeded by a maximum of 10 times

Respiratory masks of protection class FFP2/P2/N95 are suitable for work environments in which the breathing air contains substances harmful to health and capable of causing genetic alterations.

They must capture at least 94% of the particles in the air up to a size of 0.6 µm and can be used when the occupational exposure limit value reaches a maximum concentration 10 times higher. Respiratory masks of protection class FFP2 are used e.g. in the metallurgical industry or in the mining industry.

Here workers come into contact with aerosols, mists and fumes, which in the long term cause the development of respiratory diseases such as lung cancer and massively increase the risk of secondary diseases such as active lung tuberculosis.

TYPE FFP3/N100

Protection from dust, smoke and aerosol solids and liquids that are toxic and harmful to health

This protection class filters out harmful carcinogenic and radioactive substances and pathogenic microorganisms such as viruses, bacteria and fungi.

The total loss may be a maximum of 5%.

The occupational exposure limit value may be exceeded up to a maximum of 30 times higher

Respiratory masks of protection class FFP3 offer the highest possible protection against breathing air pollution. With a total loss of up to 5% and a required protection of at least 99% from particles up to 0.6 μm in size, they can also filter out toxic, carcinogenic and radioactive particles. These breathing masks can be used in work environments where the occupational exposure limit value is exceeded by up to 30 times the industry-specific value. These are used for example in the chemical industry.

Respirator Standard	Filter Capacity (removes x% diameter or larger)
FFP1 & P1	At least 80%
FFP2 & P2	At least 94%
N95	At least 95%
N99 & FFP3	At least 99%
P3	At least 99.95%
N100	At least 99.97%

WHAT ABOUT VIRUSES AND BACTERIA?

As you may have guessed, it's all about size.

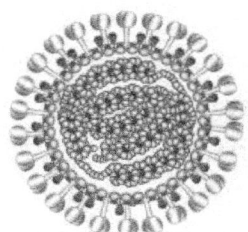 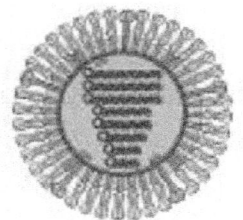

Coronavirus
0.06 - 0.14 microns
(SARS-CoV-2)

Influenza
0.08–0.12 microns

Bacteria typically have a size of about 0.45 µm, while viruses have a size in the range of 0.020-0.300 µm. This means that none of the masks discussed so far would be able to retain systems with the above dimensions.

However, if viruses and bacteria "travel" attached to colloidal particles whose size is at least 0.6 µm, then they may be blocked by FFP3 or later filtering masks. Indeed, mask manufacturers report that FFP3 type masks are good for protection against exposure to legionella (a bacterium between 0.3 and 0.9 µm wide and between 1.5 and 5 µm long) and viruses such as avian influenza, influenza A/H1N1, SARS, and tuberculosis. *However, it should be borne in mind that the filter layer of the mask tends to finish.* The mask loses its effectiveness and must be replaced. What does this mean? *That FFP masks are disposable.*

If you use them in the city, maybe during a walk, you are not defending yourself from viruses and bacteria, but simply from suspended particulate matter due to environmental contamination. When you get home, you have to throw away the mask and replace it with another one.

If you use it to defend yourself against viruses and bacteria, it is because you are not taking a walk in the middle of the exhaust fumes, but you are a healthcare worker who has to come into contact with the saliva drops of infected patients. The mask, thanks to its filtering action, prevents these pathogens from getting into our bodies.

After using, the mask must still be thrown away and replaced.

The valve on the respirators, for and against

WHAT'S THE VALVE FOR?

The protective masks FFP1, FFP2/N95 and FFP3/N100 can be equipped with valves: their presence has no effect on the filtering capacity of the device but ensures greater comfort when the mask is worn for a long time.

This is what this entails:

- the advantage of reducing breathing fatigue. Moreover, it is useful for people who have to wear the device for several hours in a row (e.g. in departments with a high risk of infection),

- the disadvantage of not filtering fumes from the wearer of the respirator. This can consequently infect others if safety distances are not observed.

Therefore, it is not recommended to use devices with VALVOLA for the general population, but also for those who work in public places (e.g. checkouts and counters in supermarkets and shops, bank and post office counters). It is also not recommended for law enforcement officials, who are often forced into close contact between colleagues (e.g. by car).

WHAT ABOUT SURGICAL MASKS?

These have nothing to do with FFP masks. While the latter protect against inhaling toxic systems, surgical masks are designed to prevent surgeons from contaminating patients' wounds during surgery. Therefore, surgical masks are used to defend the patient, not the doctor.

THE FULL MASK

Another equally important variant is the shape of the half-mask or full mask. The half-mask (or cartridge mask) covers the nose, mouth and chin (it consists of fixing straps, expiratory and inspiratory valves and a fitting for fixing the filters or air supply device) ensuring a wide field of vision. The full-face mask is used in case of risks to the eye area: for this reason, against infectious diseases such as Coronavirus - especially in high risk environments - is the only one recommended.

It consists of a harness, an eyepiece, expiratory and inspiratory valves and a fitting to fix the filters or an air supply device

Summary

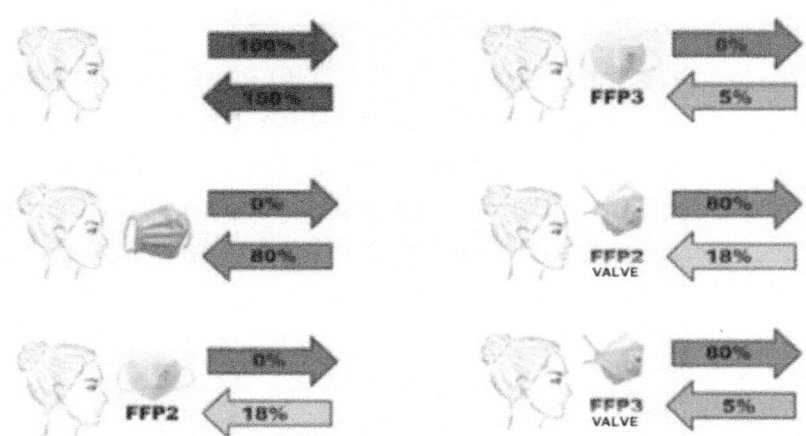

2

THE CORRECT USE OF THE PROTECTIONS

PUTTING ON OT NOT PUTTING ON THE MASK?

Let's start by clarifying the widespread WHO provisions, in apparent contradiction with what many scholars and virologists claim, the WHO recommends only to people who are sick or who exist or to health professionals to wear face masks, whereas many virologists and scholars recently advise everyone to wear them; where is the contradiction?

The good aspect is that there is no contradiction; the reason because all epidemiological virologists and doctors say to wear it, is that, with the passing of the weeks, it is becoming more and more important the contagiousness of the incubating subjects, and it is even more to the insidious contagiousness of the asymptomatic subjects.

Coronavirus is among us, in the people we meet at the supermarket, at the newsstand, in the pharmacy, we could be ourselves to release it in the air.

However, everyone thinks that coronavirus patients are always "the others". It is estimated that an infected person can infect nor 18 others, only during the incubation period. Imagine then what can happen in case of an asymptomatic subjects for the duration of the pathology.

It is important to know that the virus survives and spreads in the air only inside saliva droplets; there are two types of saliva droplets: a very fine aerosol put with breathing, that evaporates after a few seconds killing any coronavirus inside it, and larger droplets emitted with a cough or talking that travel a distance of about one meter, a meter and a half before settling on the ground by gravity.

Therefore, risk is very high when a sick person is a short distance, because the emitted particles can reach directly and quickly our oral olfactory ocular mucous membranes; for this reason, there are two precautions that have asked us to respect: avoiding people so that the sulphurous air is put with breathing and vapors can't reach us, and respecting the interpersonal distance of 3/5 feet so that even the largest particles emitted fall to the ground on objects before reaching us.

WHEN TO WEAR THE MASK?

In the open air with a few people and distances even greater than 6 feet it is not necessary to wear surgical masks or FFP3; for example, when you are in line at the supermarket, in the street, driving your own car or if you walk alone do not waste them.

At the contrary, in situation of closed environments with still air and distances greater than 3 feet, like inside a supermarket it is important that everyone wear masks.

We should not be afraid of closed-air common spaces such as corridors or elevators, because even if a sick person has passed through them before us, there are no more contagious particles in the air when we arrive, the WHO virologists' statements are not contradictory; the first claims that only sick people should wear facial protection, the second one that we should all consider ourselves sick because of the incubation period and asymptomatic cases.

That is why we all have to wear facial protection in the right way and in the right situations.

LET'S TALK ABOUT SERGICAL MASKS AND FFP3.

Caution cover the nose mouth with a mask serves to prevent the droplets from moving away from the diseased subject infecting the next one does not serve to avoid our contagion. In this regard it is necessary to open a parenthesis on the most diffused type of masks, that is the surgical ones and the FFP3 masks.

The first ones have a very effective filtering capacity for the outgoing air and are able to hold most of the particles emitted with a cough with breathing or with dialogue.

On the contrary, the FFP3 masks filter very well the incoming air while the outgoing ones are almost not at all; in the front part of the mask there is no filter but a valve that lets out the air completely unfiltered. To summarize, we can say that the correct choice to go out of the house and go shopping or buy drugs in the pharmacy is the surgical mask because we always must consider ourselves potentially contagious and we must not transmit the disease to the others.

Let's use the FFP3 masks to the healthcare staff; there are few of them in circulation and they are the ones who need to protect themselves 100% from people who are certainly sick and it is no coincidence that they wear goggles.

THE IMPORTANCE OF SAFETY GLASSES

Here is another very important point: the virus enters our body through the oral olfactory mucous membranes but also through the ocular mucous membranes, so it is completely useless to wear protective masks such as FFP3 if you do not use protective goggles too.

Moreover, it is essential that everyone wear surgical masks so as to emit air that is not contagious and make it unnecessary to use protective goggles.

HOW THE VIRUS SURVIVES ON SURFACES?

Someone will be wondering why a virus that almost does not survive in the air is able to do so for one, two or three days on surfaces.

When it falls on the ground or ends up on objects especially in public places, like handles of supermarket trolleys, it meets an organic substrate invisible to the naked eye in which it survives for a long time from which it is protected.

THE WAY TO USE THE MASKS

The reasons why the WHO suggests only sick patients to wear the mask and also why if it is done incorrectly, it is more dangerous than protective. Most of all if it regards a healthy person, the risk of getting infected by incorrect use of the mask is very high.

THE SURGICAL MASK

Here we talk about this light, simple and effective mask. After two or three hours it should be replaced because the water vapor, put with breathing, is the viral load that may be present inside it and that compromise its effectiveness.

So masks are a valuable ally but it is important to take care of them and to use them at the right time to not waste them.

Wear a mask only when it's really necessary so in situations where you suspect the interpersonal distance can be reduced to less than one meter.

Before wearing it, wash your hands for at least 30 seconds rubbing well or with an alcoholic solution, when you put it on your face you must stretch it well on the nose and chin and you must shape the nasal iron so that it adheres well to the face.

While you are wearing it, never touch the external part even to fix it better, never lower it under the chin to make a phone call because you may lack air or for any other reason because both the external and the internal part must always be considered contaminated.

When you take it off by yourself by the elastic bands, dispose it in a plastic bag well closed inside the rubbish. After using it wash your hands with soap for 30-40 seconds or use a 75% alcohol solution. All other important hygiene rules to be respected.

The hygiene rules to be respected are:

Wash your hands with soap and water even for 30-40 50 seconds massaging well or otherwise use alcoholic solutions at 75/80%, remember that at concentrations greater than 90-95 these are very ineffective.

You always have to sneeze and cough in the elbow socket.

Gatherings must be avoided.

Interpersonal distances of 3 feet even 6 feet must be respected.

You should not touch your face, unfortunately we all do it inadvertently even three times a minute but they risk contaminating our oral or olfactory or ocular mucous membranes.

I RECOMMEND IF YOU ONLY HAVE ONE MASK

Last but not least, we face the chronic shortage that many people do not have masks at all or in the luckiest cases they have only one.

So what I'm about to give you is advice, not an advice on things that normally should never be done but something more important.

The indications are as follows: the masks, after being used, must be considered contaminated on the outside as well as on the inside, so they must be handled only by elastic bands and must be hung so as not to contaminate any surface; if you have a few but more than one do not use the same mask several times during the same day but wait for the next day, because if the virus is present is dead or in any case the viral load has been greatly reduced.

When you return home put the masks under the sun and, if you have the opportunity, turn them several times during the day in order to disinfect both sides; UV rays of the Sun have the characteristic of damaging the DNA of viruses and bacteria as happens also for our skin when they cause cancer. After being used, the masks should then be hung or placed carefully on the concave side; do not put them in your pocket or bag because they could contaminate objects with which they come into contact.

3

HOW TO CREATE AN EFFECTIVE HOMEMADE MASK

Given for good reason that the face mask works to protect against contagion, and even if they have a minimal effectiveness they are always better than nothing, then let's try to make them at home. Unfortunately, surgical masks are also difficult to find online and in pharmacies, so it's worth making them yourself.

Here are some do-it-yourself solutions:

1 Make the mask with baking paper

All you need to build an anti-virus mask with baking paper is elastic bands and staples. You fold the baking paper in a certain way and then you can wear it using the elastic bands pinned on the paper, to be effective you need to use two layers of baking paper, otherwise it remains too light and vulnerable.

What do I need?

•　　baking paper, not just any baking paper, but a baking paper that does not let the water pass through if wet; to test the quality of the paper just create a basin with the baking paper and pour it in some water; if the water does not come out, leave it like this for a while 'time to decant and if after half an hour the paper holds without passing water on the other side this means that it is suitable.

•　　scissors

•　　a stapler and its pins

•　　elastic by the meter but you can also use the office elastic or a normal hair band

Proceeding:

For woman we take the measure of 25cm (9"7/8), for man we take the measure of 30cm (11"7/8) lengthwise: just cut straight enough to form a rectangle which will be longer in the paper direction of the roll.

Creates from the folds of about 1,6cm (5/8) each to form an accordion

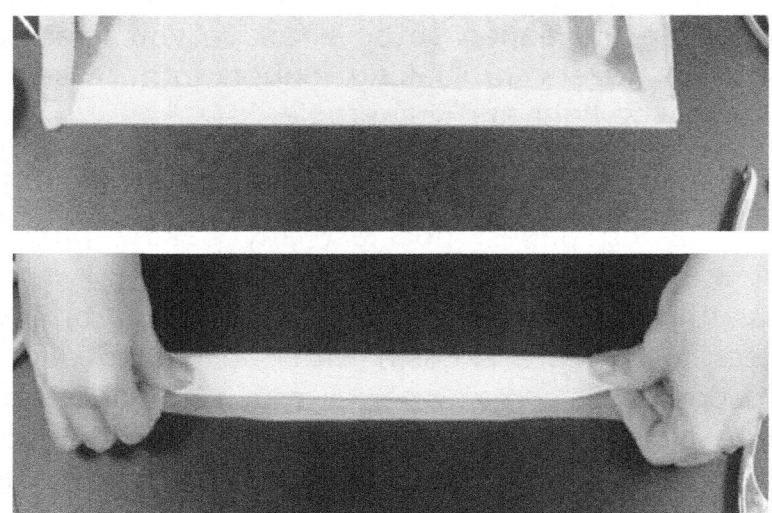

Fold in about 3cm (1"1/4) x 3cm (1"1/4) and with the stapler lock it leaving a loop wide enough to insert the elastic inside.

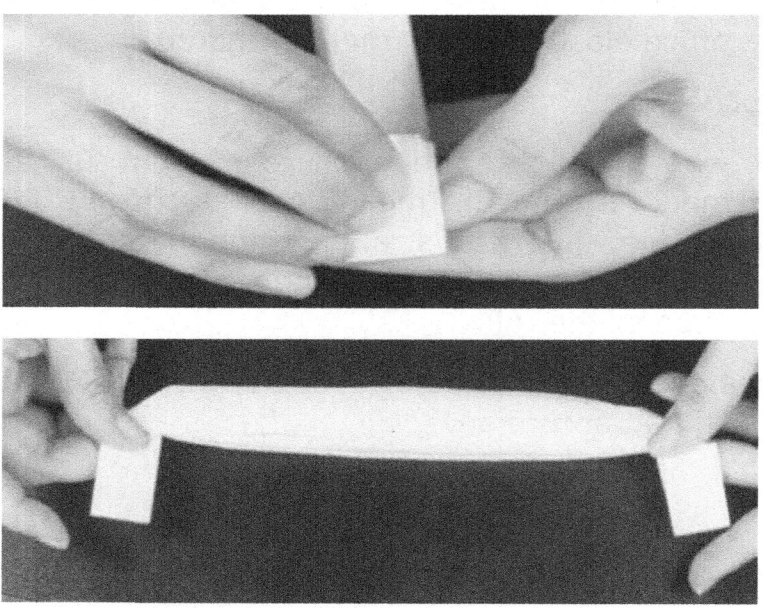

Insert the rubber band and do the same thing on the other side and then stop well with the stapler, be careful to leave the staples of the stapler on the outside.

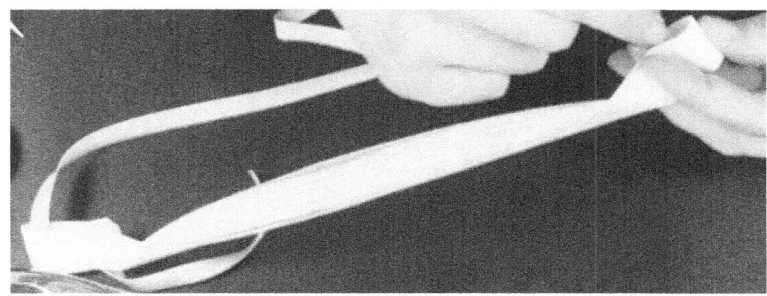

Slowly widen what will be our mask and close it to see the folds, then once closed we pass inside our elastic band.

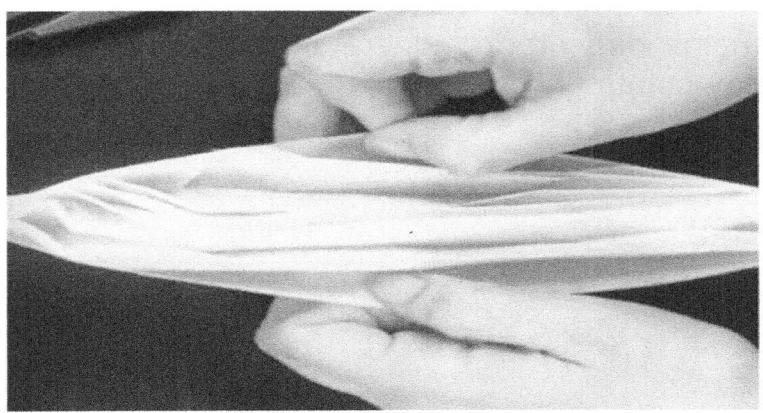

Our mask is ready to be used! If the elastic bands are slow, just tighten them further.

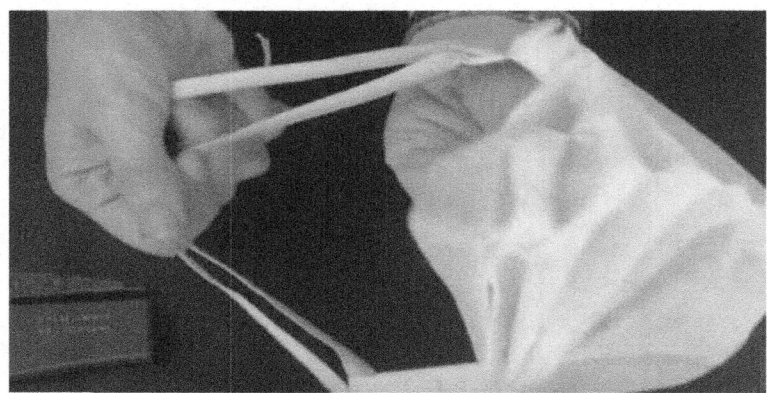

To test its effectiveness, do the breathability test: stand two cm in front of a mirror and breathe, if the paper is good the mirror should not fog.

If you want a higher degree of protection, use two layers of paper.

The problem with this type of mask is that it remains difficult to adhere to the face, leaving many points uncovered.

2. Masks with waterproof mats or crossbars for babies

Here is an idea of practical and fast DIY masks suitable especially for those who cannot sew.

These masks are made with waterproof mats such as those used for dogs and cats, but also waterproof crossbars that are used for babies or the elderly are good.

What you need:

- a sanitary mat for animals or a crossbar...
- stapler
- scissors
- optional paper belt (to be used to prevent cellulose from coming out)
- common elastics or alternatively use underwear elastics

Proceeding:

Open the mat, this material has the peculiarity that it is composed of two materials: one external smooth water-repellent that serves to block water particles and a breathable layer that is the inner part (the latter is a hypoallergenic and soft fabric in contact with the skin and has an inner layer that is pure cellulose).

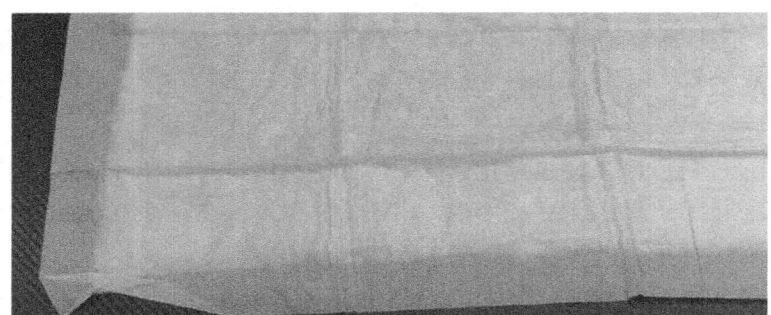

Cut the outer edge of only water-repellent material that we do not need, the idea is to cut strips about 20cm (7"7/8) high and about 50cm (19"3/4) long

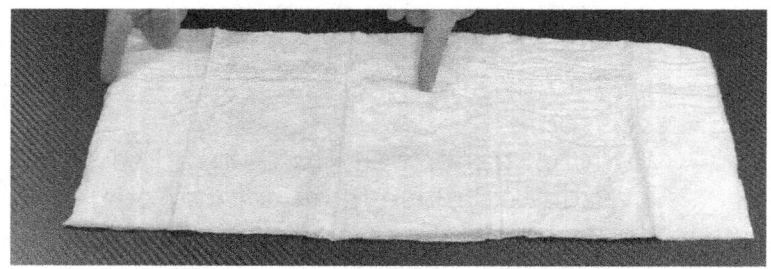

Divide into two parts in order to obtain a distance of 25cm (9"7/8) (this is more or less the useful measure for an average face)

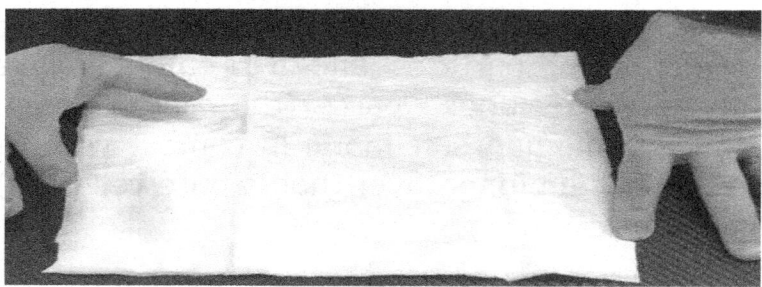

Take a side and fold it like in the picture

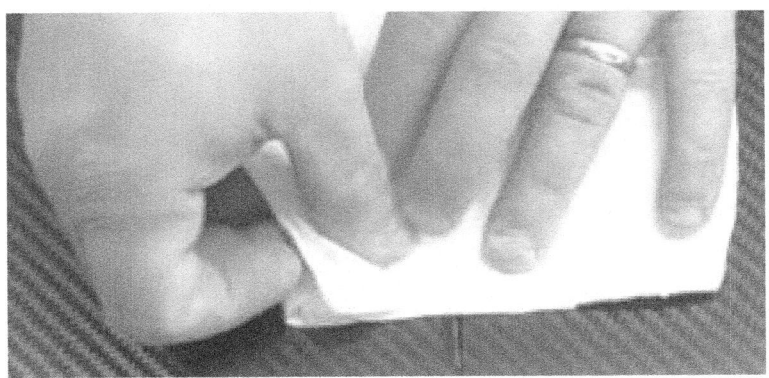

Insert a rubber band and lock it in at least 3 points with the stapler.

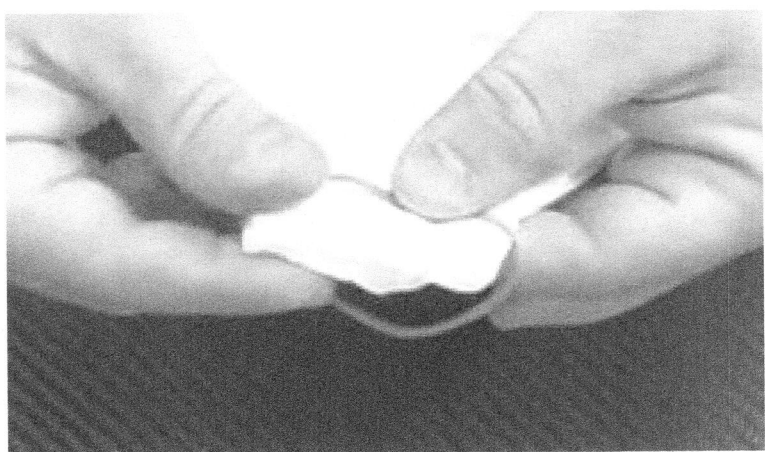

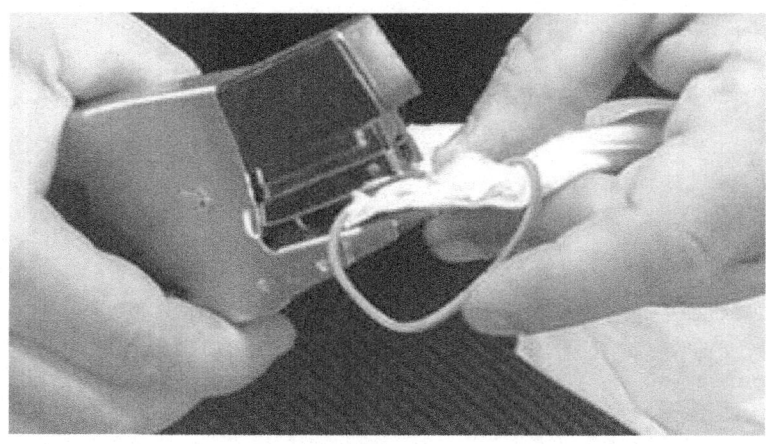

Do the same operation on the other side, paying attention to the points that must be facing outwards, even if you notice that the cellulose applied to the edge of the paper mask comes out

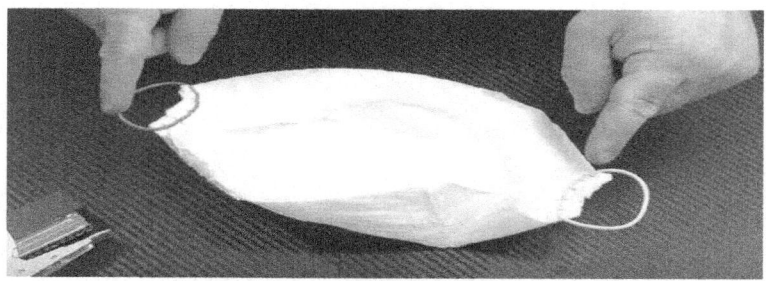

We have our mask that we're going to model on the face and put rubber bands behind the ears. (if you have used the elastic bands on your underwear you can leave it long enough and tie it around your head)

3. Fabric surgical masks

These masks can be made in cotton, or in stain-resistant cotton (the stain-resistant fabric prevents the external liquid droplets from passing through the mask and therefore coming into contact with our mouth). They are breathable masks, suitable for every size thanks to the elastic to be placed behind the ears.

They are considered personal protective equipment, but are not intended to equate the masks with the ffp2 or ffp3 filters, but rather to provide personal protective equipment in the absence of any other device. These masks can be made in many colors and we can match them to the color of the dress we are wearing; then, the cotton masks are really useful regardless of any health emergency, because they can come very comfortable when we simply are cold and we want to protect our interlocutors from any bacilli or bacteria that we may transmit.

It is necessary:

- 100% cotton fabric because it is machine washable at high temperatures and can also be added hygienic if necessary.
- scissors
- elastic from 0,3cm (1/8) to 0,6cm (1/4) (or what you have available)
- needle and thread or sewing machine
- pins
- chalk

Proceeding:

Prepare two 20cm (7"7/8) squares and two 20cm (7"7/8) rubber bands.

Draw with a chalk of the 2,20cm (7/8) lines on the right and left side from the upper and lower edges of the two pieces respectively as shown below

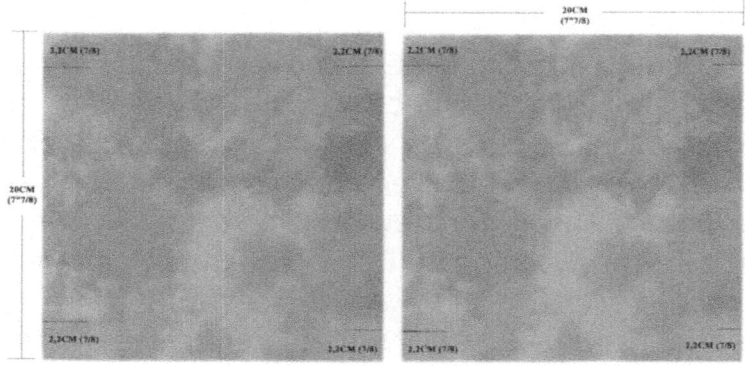

Place one end of the elastic on the right upper side of the fabric on the right upper part and stop it with a pin, take the other end of the elastic and stop it on the right lower part.

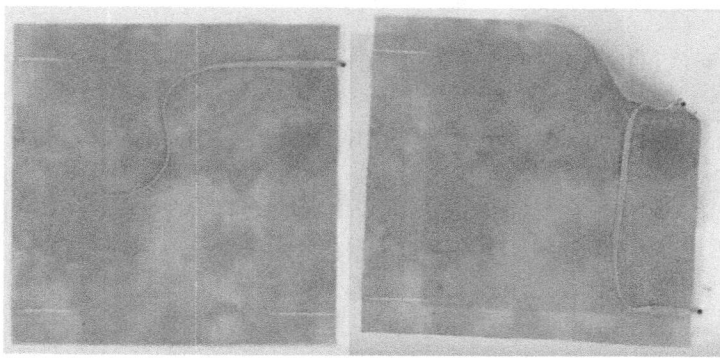

Do the usual operation on the other side too, take the other piece of square and overlap it directly on top and match the chalk line, try to lock the top piece with the pins already positioned without moving the elastic.

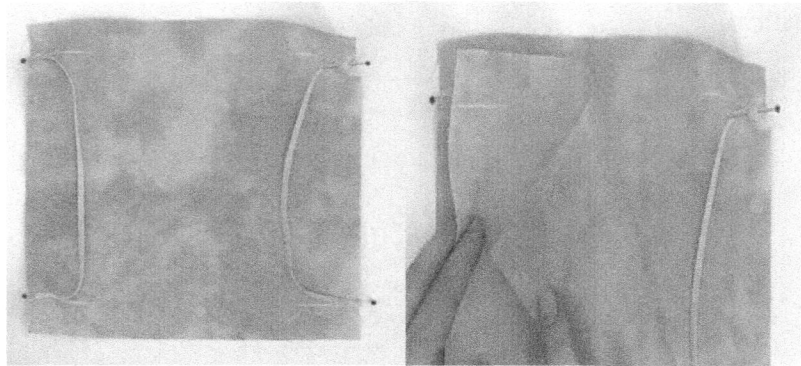

Insert the pins in the marked stitches (A) and proceed with the straight stitching with a margin of 0,6cm (1/4) following the figure below being careful not to sew the part between the two marked pins (not sew), the part you didn't sew will be used to turn up the mask itself. Once the mask has been turned upside down, proceed with ironing.

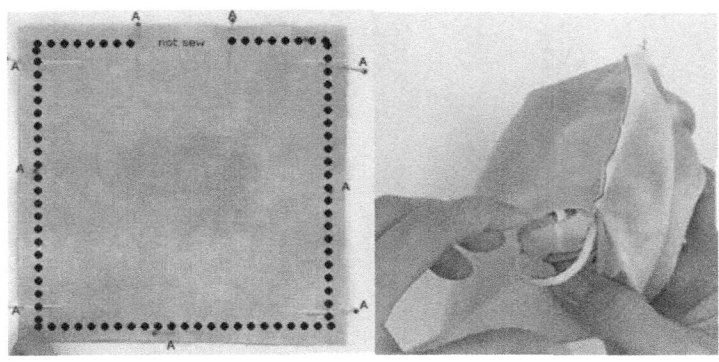

Run six horizontal lines from the top

The first one at 4cm (1"5/8), the second one at 3cm (1"1/4), the third one at 1,6cm (5/8), the fourth one at 3cm (1"1/4), the fifth one at 1,6 cm (5/8) and the sixth one 3cm (1"1/4) as follows

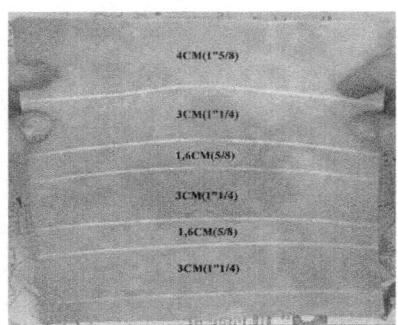

Now fold the first line on the second one as in the picture, take the second line and fold it on the third one and the third one on the fourth one.

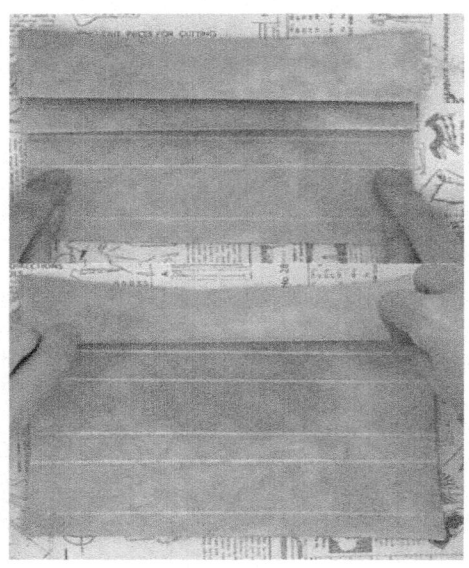

Once all the folds have been made, iron the surface so as to fix them and insert the pins to lock them, at this point proceed with the stitching of the entire edge.

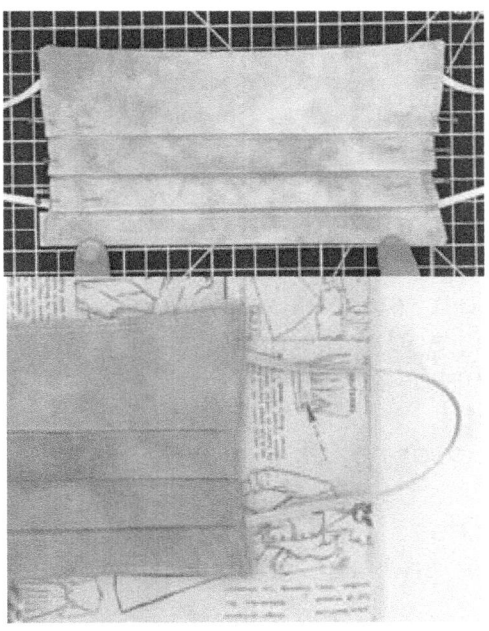

Here's the cotton elasticated ear mask with pleats

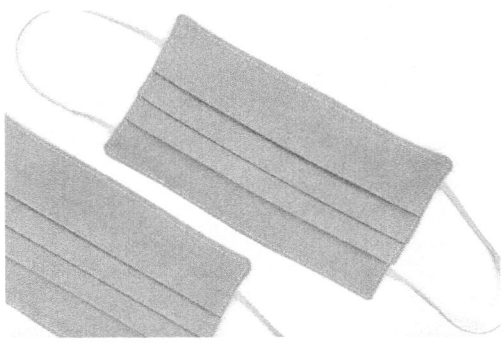

4. DIY masks in neoprene, crackle rubber or jersey

Finally, this is a DIY mask model with holes for the ears and therefore without elastic bands. It can be sewn by machine but also by hand and the material with which it can be made must be elastic of its own.

It is necessary:

- a piece of neoprene (better known as scuba fabric), crackle rubber (the softest or thinnest one) or even jersey as long as it is strong and resistant.
- scissors
- pencil
- a sheet of paper
- ruler
- Brooches
- needle and thread or sewing machine

Procedure:

To execute the pattern, draw a polygon with the measurements below and draw the mask as shown in the picture

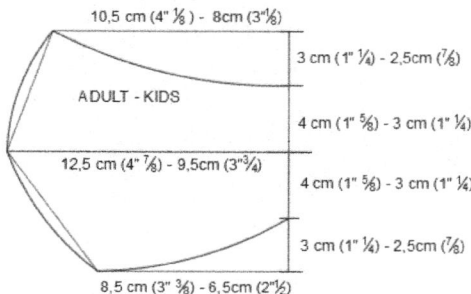

10,5 cm (4" ⅛) - 8cm (3"⅛)

3 cm (1" ¼) - 2,5cm (⅞)

ADULT - KIDS

4 cm (1" ⅝) - 3 cm (1" ¼)

12,5 cm (4" ⅞) - 9,5cm (3"¾)

4 cm (1" ⅝) - 3 cm (1" ¼)

3 cm (1" ¼) - 2,5cm (⅞)

8,5 cm (3" ⅜) - 6,5cm (2"½)

Draw two parallel lines from zero point one to the right side at 4cm (1"5/8)" and the other to the left side 1cm (3/8).

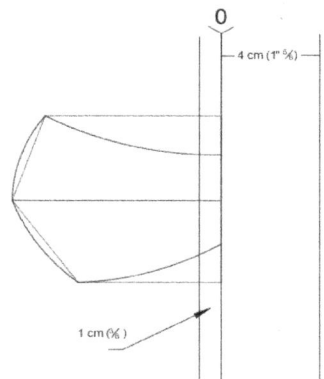

Extend the horizontal center line to the right parallel line and join points 1-2 and 3-4.

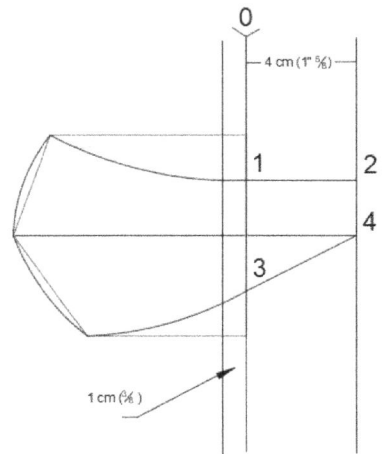

Inside the pattern, draw a figure keeping a distance of 1,5cm (5/8) from the upper, lower and right edges while arriving at the left parallel line as shown below, after drawing a parallel line at 0.6cm (1/4)" on the left side.

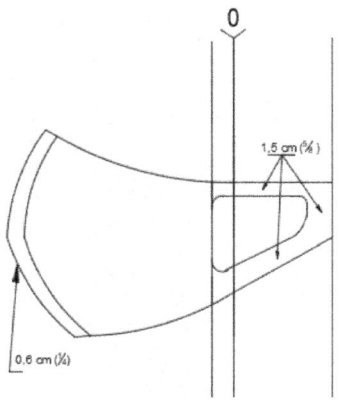

At this point cut out with the scissors

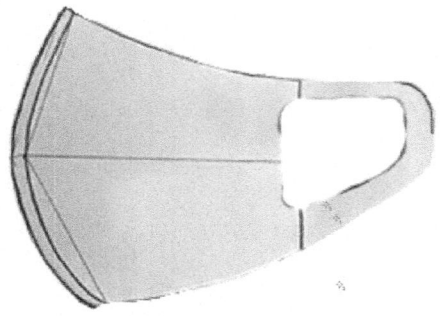

Take the material you have chosen and put it in duplicate, place the model on it, mark it with a pencil and pin it with pins.

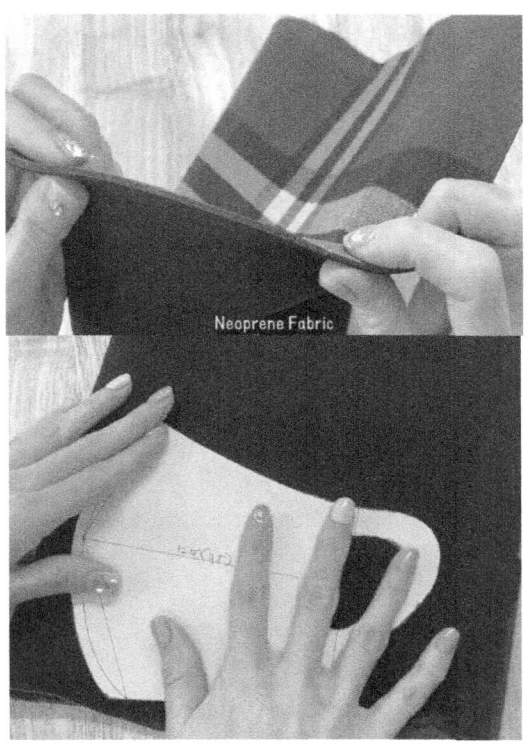

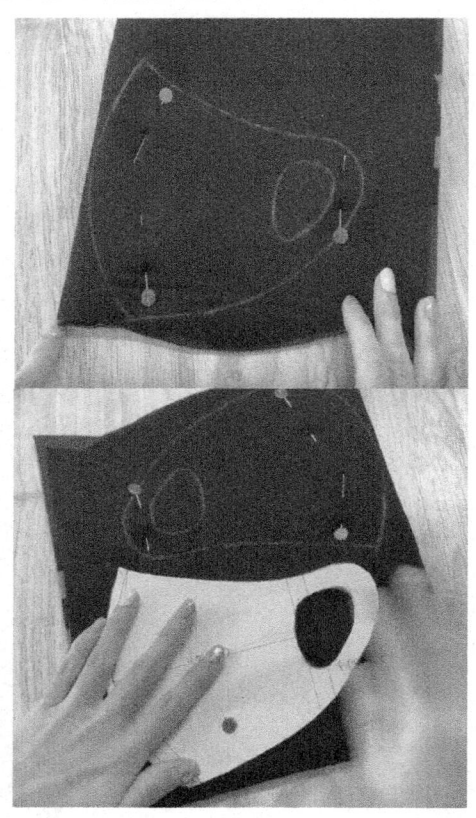

Cut the fabric and mate it

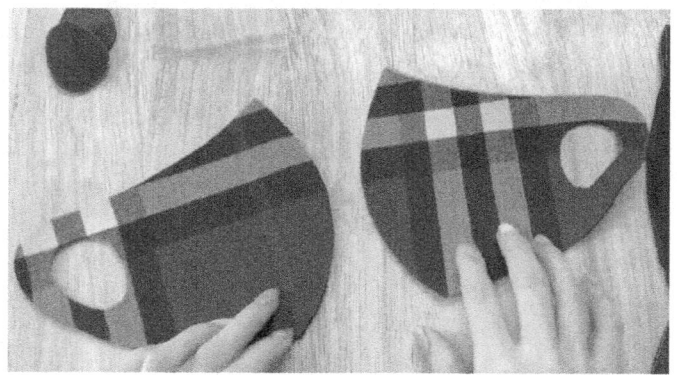

Sew along the right side first in a linear fashion and then in a zigzag pattern

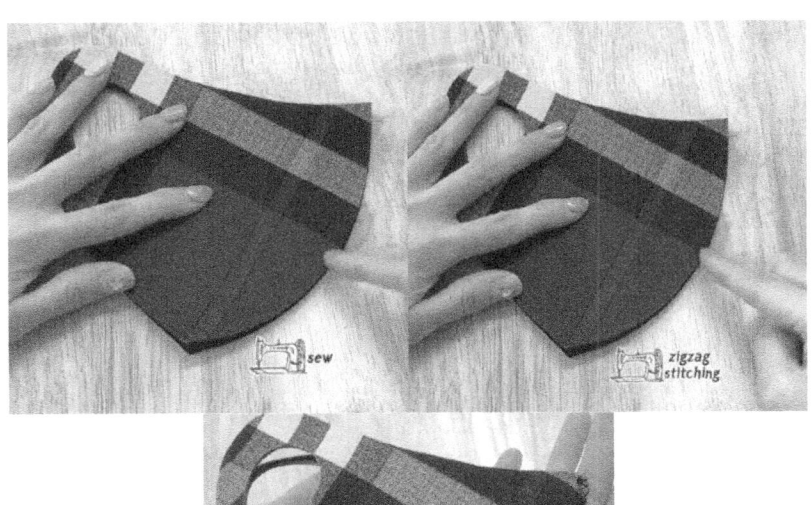

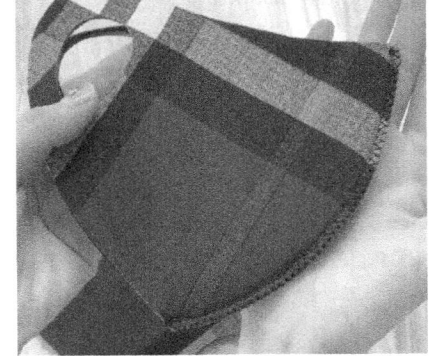

The mask is ready to be worn

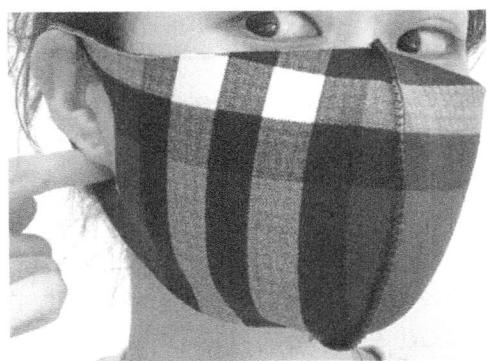

5. Fabric masks with filter pocket

This type of mask with interchangeable filter for young and old requires the sewing machine. To make it we will recycle materials that we have already found in the house.

It is necessary:

- a scissor
- pins
- a thread
- an old cotton shirt or other remnants of cloth always in cotton
- a sewing machine
- elastic bands or alternatively you can also cut a strip from a stocking
- a sheet of baking paper
- a team
- flexible closure of a package (optional)
- sterile bandages or disposable wipes

Proceeding:

Let's start by drawing the pattern: draw a rectangle with one side of 15cm (5" 7/8) and the other one of 12cm (4"3/4). Then, divide the half starting from the left side, mark a point at 3,5cm (1"3/8). On the right side instead starting from the upper vertex go down 4,5cm (1"3/4), from the lower vertex of the right side go up 3,5cm (1"3/8). Then connect all the stitches, on the right side draw a parallel line at a distance of 3cm (1"1/4) and add 1 cm (3/8)" of seam.

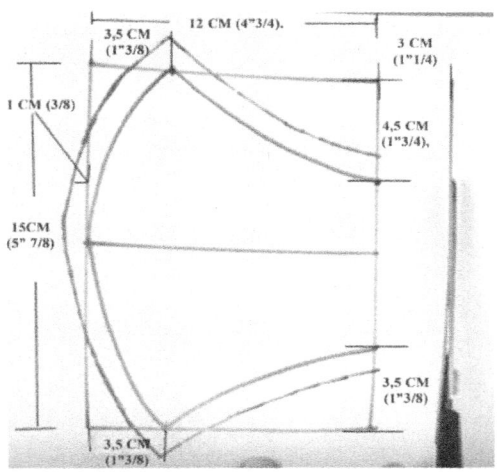

Cut out along the parallel line on the right side and then fold it 1cm (3/8) to the left side and then fold it again following the line and cut out along the outer line

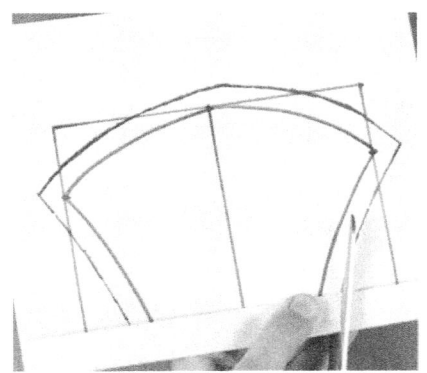

To make the pattern of the inside of the template, cover the top of the pattern on the baking paper, draw at a distance of 2,5cm (1") a line parallel to the center line of the pattern paper

and add another 1,60cm (5/8)", folded and cut out.

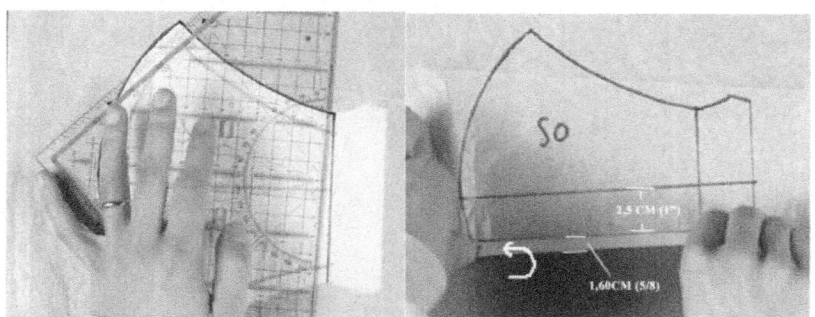

Don't forget to redraw also the pattern of the lower part that you will make in the same way, here the upper and lower part are ready.

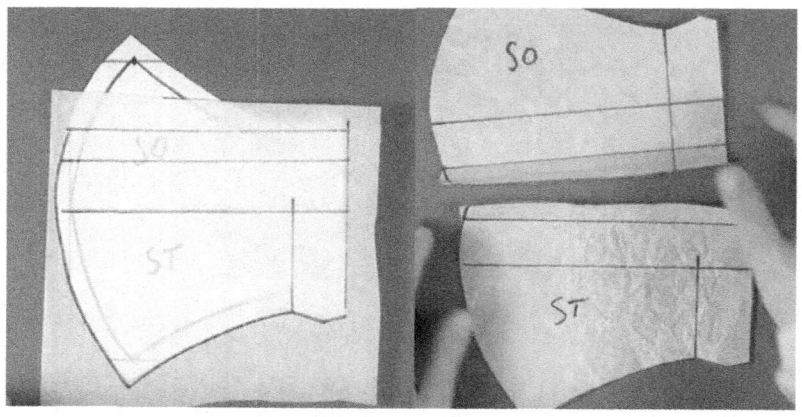

Here we report the measurements for the children's pattern here

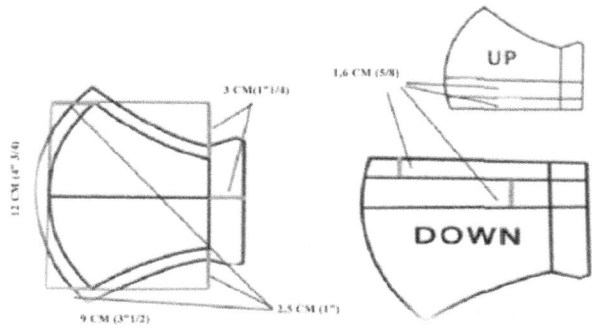

Now arrange your fabric in duplicate, staple and cut out

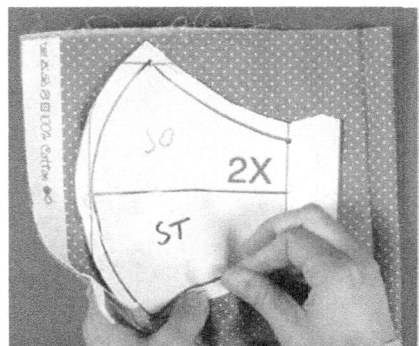

Mark all the notches by making a small cut on the fabric.

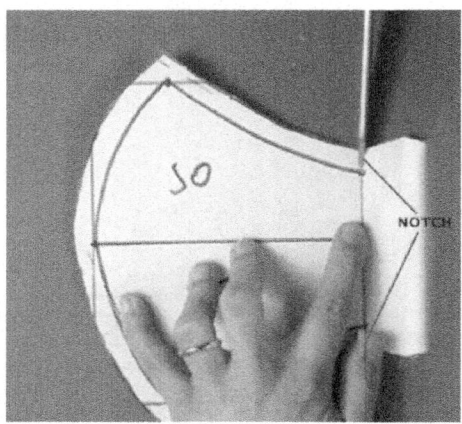

Place the straight stitch with the straight stitch, staple and sew, finish with a zigzag stitch and cut off the excess fabric.

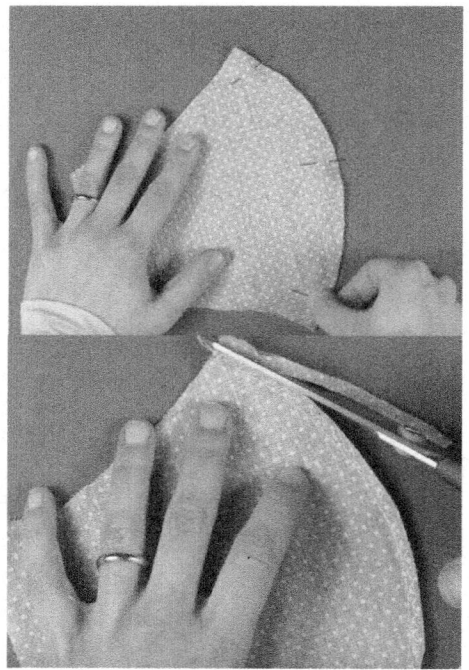

Now cut out the inner parts of the mask and mark all the notches as a small cut and you will have a total of four pieces here also place straight on the straight and sew first with a straight stitch then with a zigzag stitch

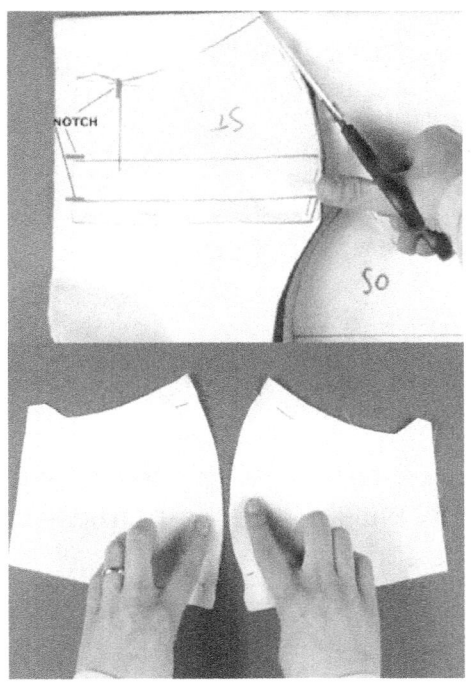

Shorten those seams here too and make a stitching to fix the central seam on all the pieces of the mask.

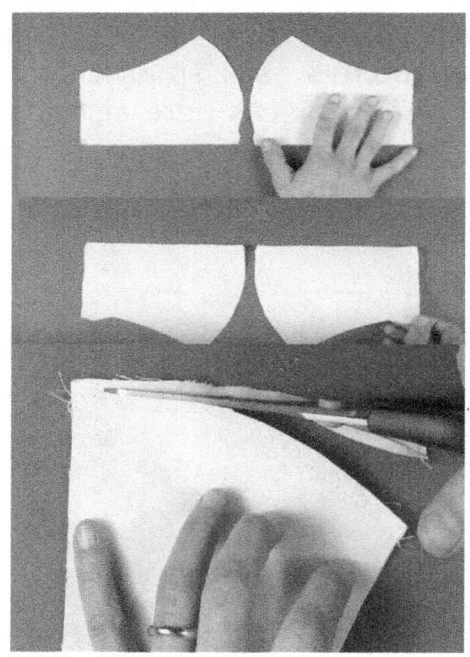

Now take the inner pieces of the mask the marked notch will be the point until you have to repeat it for beading

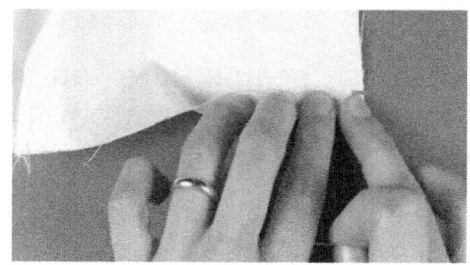

Stapled and sewn

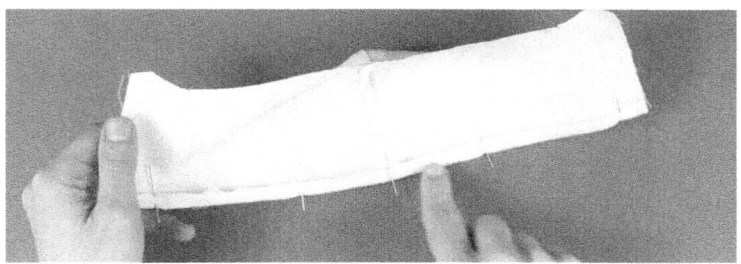

When the edges are sewn together the two internal parts matching the notches

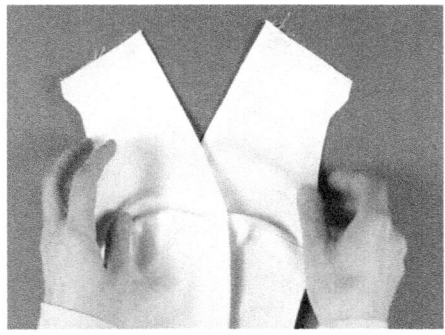

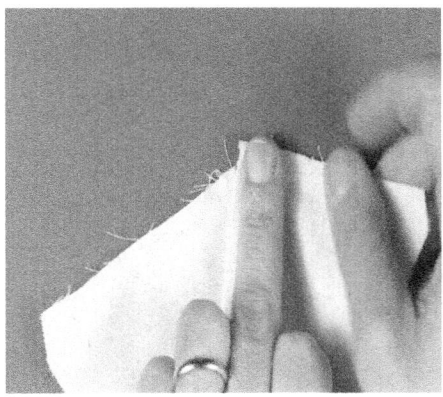

Fix them with a 0.6cm (1/4) seam

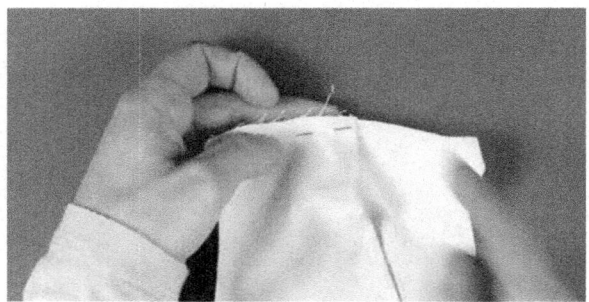

Now you can sew the outside and the inside of the mask together, put straight with the straight stitch and sew it

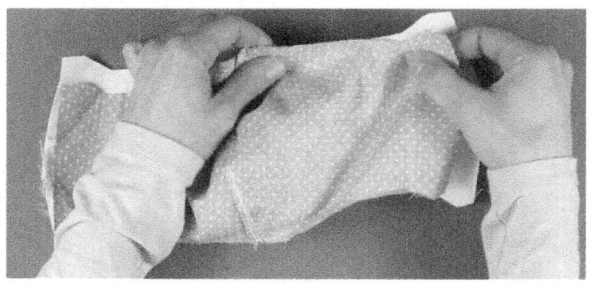

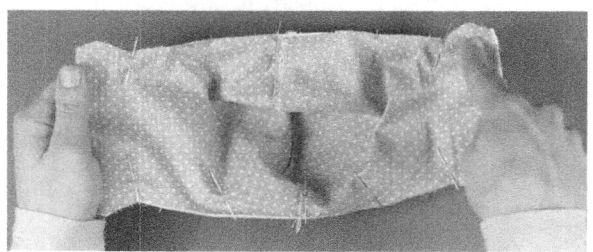

When you get to the corners, leave the needle down on the sewing machine, lift the presser foot, turn the fabric and sew, shorten the seams 0.6cm (1/4) in the corners and cut the seam to 45 degrees, turn it all taking care to fold well the inner seams in the corners

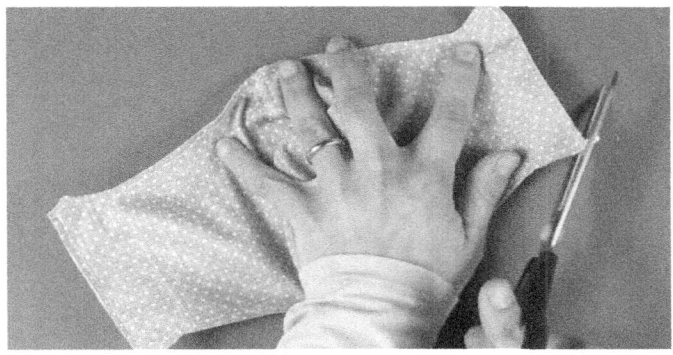

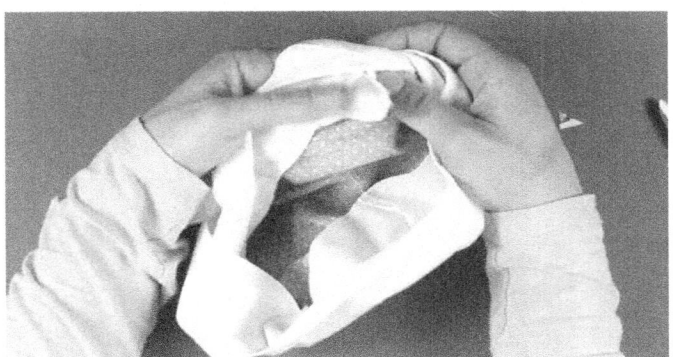

Now is the time to insert the flexible part for the nose this step is optional if you want the mask to fit perfectly insert the flexible closure between the two layers of fabric and set it with sewn pins

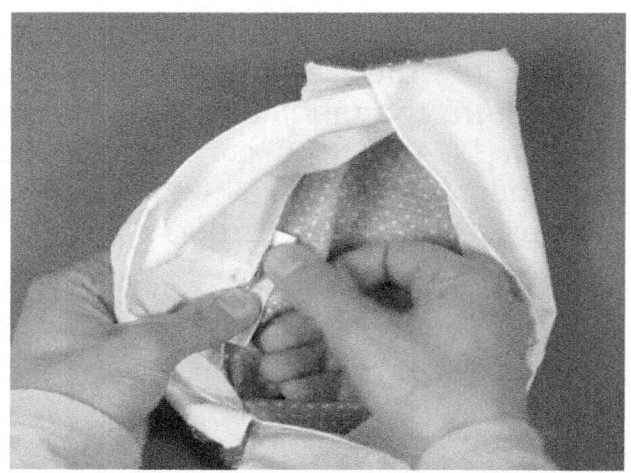

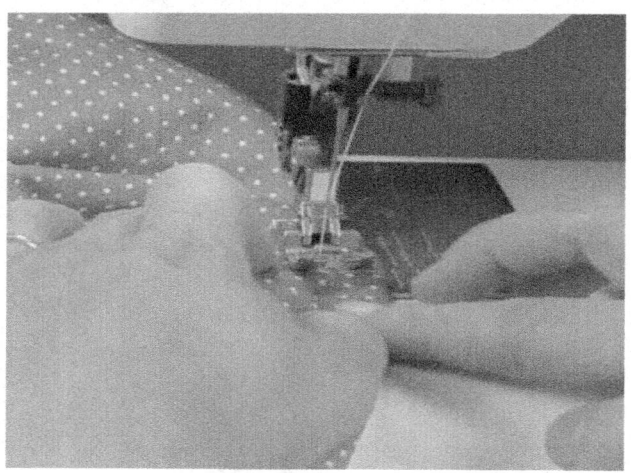

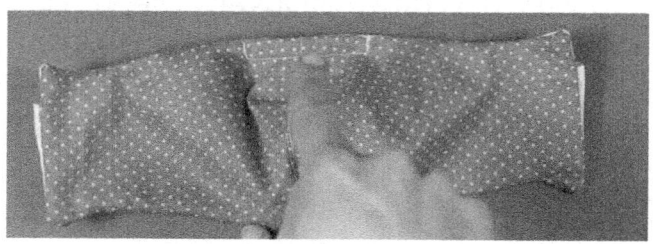

Now stitch a stitch over the entire edge of the mask, fold 1,5cm (5/8) one end and secure with two parallel seams.

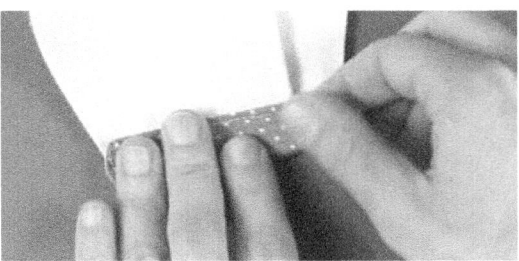

When you're done, insert the rubber band into the tunnel with the help of a safety pin...

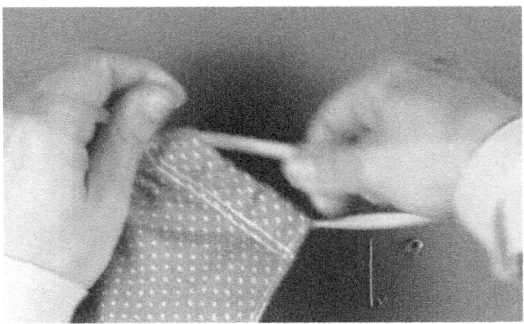

Try the mask and determine the right length of your elastic, then hide the nose of the elastic inside the tunnel, finally cut the filter of the right size and insert it into the pocket and the mask is complete.

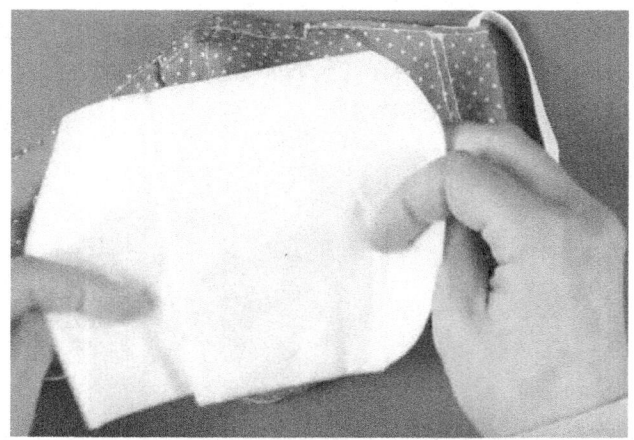

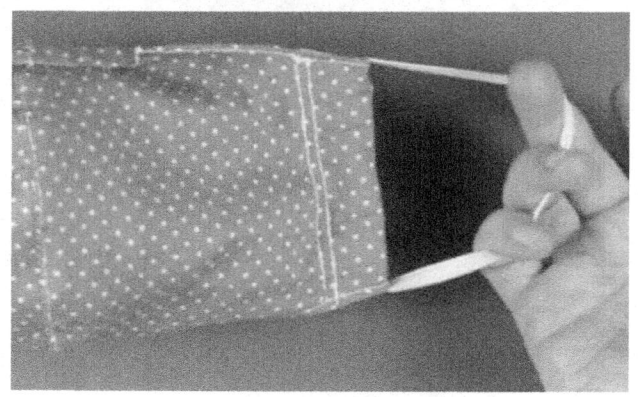

Made in the USA
Monee, IL
17 February 2021